Copyright © 2023 H.B.Giat

hbgiat2023@gmail.com

2 T1D
A FAMILY TALE

H.B. GIAT

ILLUSTRATIONS BY Maria Dronfort

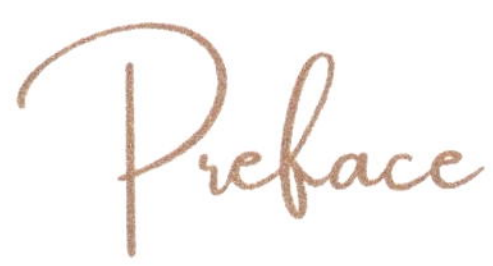

This book is dedicated to all of the children, teenagers and adults who have been diagnosed with Type 1 Diabetes, and their families. Hence its somewhat strange title. I guess it feels like we are all sharing the same family name, and I knew that by choosing T1D as part of the book's title, all family members who come across it will pick it up straightaway.

This book is essentially an autobiography, my family tale, and our way of living with T1D. All the characters and facts are very much real—well, except for the obvious ones...

Being a parent to two diabetic kids, I've always wanted to write my own memoir, but I didn't really think I'd have the time, until now.

When I first introduced the idea of writing a book, telling our story, my children were ecstatic—it took me by complete surprise. They were encouraging me, pushing me to do so. So I knew the timing was right and I must accept my call. A gift to our family as we mark the first decade.

Here I am now, just a few months later, feeling happy and liberated. The writing process had served us all as an ongoing deep cleansing session.

Of course, I had to revisit all of the dark places I've tried so hard to bury deep down inside. Reconnect with so many emotions and worries I've tried to leave behind. Tears were very much part of it, and I had to make sure they only appear when my kids were out at school.

Before Covid-19 interrupted our mundane lives, we used to spend six months of the year surrounded by the beautiful English countryside, especially around the Cotswolds. It is the area's extraordinary beauty that has helped heal our hearts, and that is the reason I have decided to write our story as a family of squirrels living in the English countryside. Firstly, as a means of protecting my children's identities, but mainly to give our story a different dimension—not only one of burden and tears, so to speak. And lastly, because my children are very, well, naughty! And they are all over the place. God bless them.

I should also note that it is the real Mr. Daddypaw who first came out with the "Paw family" notion many years ago. All four of us have a Paw added to our names. So, if your name is, for example, Freddie, you become Freddiepaw.

A decade has passed since my first child was diagnosed with T1D. He was only 25 months old. Three years later, his sister was diagnosed too, also at 25 months old. Although I feel more confident and definitely more experienced, it is far from being easy. I had to forget about my career as a lawyer; I had to put my life and my needs on hold. I had to adapt to a new reality and become a nurse 24/7 without a break. But I should not really complain—I am no different from any parent caring for a child with a chronic disease. Burden, stress, worries, and sleepless nights are part of our everyday life.

After my son was first diagnosed with T1D we were completely lost; I felt like a zombie and there was nothing to hold onto. My heart was shattered into million pieces. I didn't want to let go. I didn't want to drift away from my baby's perfect health. But we had no choice—bit by bit we started to channel our way up the best we could. Our goal is of course a life free of T1D, but until we all get there, it doesn't mean we can't have happy and fulfilling lives.

While T1D has its many challenges, I think it is also a matter of how one chooses to deal with it (after the first blow to the head): look for the best options available, for the best way forward. Even if everything seems to be bad, we must try to find one positive thing, no matter how small or trivial. Like, for instance, keeping a healthy diet. We must always try and stay positive even when we don't feel up to it. It is very easy to be consumed by negativity. In my case, I had two toddlers to take care of, so it wasn't really an option—I had to keep on going.

Always look for the light in the darkness. It will be there. Hold on to it no matter how frail it might seem, until the glorious day arrives and Type One Diabetes is eliminated forever from the book of chronic diseases. Gone and no more.

The day will come. It is getting closer every day, thanks to the efforts of many devoted doctors and researchers all around the globe.

I wish you and your families very happy, healthy, and content lives.

I hope you will enjoy reading this book, I promise it is funny and happy and not all sad.

With love xxx

p/s – you are more than welcome to leave a comment or tell us your story and /or your thoughts at t1dpawfamily@gmail.com

The Paw Family

This is a tale of a squirrel family, my remarkable family. My name is Mamapaw, a title which was given to me by Mr. Daddypaw, in honor of our two extraordinary, wondrous, marvelous, super -active -never tired, extremely intense, funny, clever squirrels—Leopaw and Kalipaw, and we are the Paw family.

We live in Wickershaw Way, a hidden spot in the beautiful English Cotswolds, where everything is surrounded by an outstanding nature. Just a short trip down to the next river or stream, through the evergreen woods, or the many gorgeous picturesque gardens is so uplifting and soul healing and so very much recommended. We have a lovely little cottage, Woods Lane No. 6, up the stairs. Although very small, it is our own kingdom decorated with all of the treasures we have collected through the years. Leaves (especially autumn leaves with their splendid colors), pinecones big and small, sticks and stones, and all sorts of shells from all around the globe – well, at least parts of it. Some we have collected during a trip to Cancun or the Cayman Islands, some were picked around the Mediterranean and some came from the beautiful beaches of Cornwall. I am so proud of my two little squirrels, who, just like me, have learned to enjoy picking up these organic magical treasures, and appreciate their wondrous existence.

Our house is indeed very cozy and warm – too warm if you ask Mr. Daddypaw (and Leopaw) but I just can't help it! I can't stand the freezing cold… Gives me the shivers! I suppose the fact that the kitchen is always busy and ready to receive hungry little mouths, and the AGA is working nonstop, filling up the air with tasty baked fluffy dreams, is adding a little bit of extra heat and excitement. If you come over for a visit, you might feel you are walking inside an English fairy tale, with Halloween, Xmas, and Easter décor all year round, lots of candles and flowers everywhere, and, of course, there is the extra-large fireside. Well, I can go on forever and talk about the bits and pieces around our house, but I am pretty sure most of you will find it simply boring.

Long before I met Mr. Daddypaw, I used to work in the busy bustling city, Squirrelton Bush. Much like the city, I too was trying to catch my own breath, working days to nights in a gloomy office at *Acron & Balut Solicitors Ltd*, rushing between one court and another, meeting with clients, preparing my cases, answering hysterical telephone calls, reading piles and piles of legal documents, and on occasions comforting my heartbroken secretary who has lost—again—the love of her life. "But this time it was the real one!"… Oh it was exhausting, I tell you that. I always felt I was running around my tail in hyperventilation. Dropping onto my bed at the end of another day, only to find the next morning a new pile of cases sitting on my office desk, staring at me with a mocking "face" as I approach them with horror.

You can understand how happy I was when I met Mr. Daddypaw and left my hectic career behind. Only for a short time, I thought. The timing was perfect. I mean, I needed a time-out to remind myself it's okay to get off the fast track, find a new direction, new ideas and dreams, and be the boss of my own time. It was so refreshing not having to repeat my footsteps every day over and over again. I would wake up in my tiny apartment after a long night's sleep, minus the annoying sound of the alarm clock, spirit so high it was like picking up a new book every morning, curious about the tale about to be told and the adventures awaiting.

A new beginning it was, and while I have never much left the lawyer behind me—you know how it is when you have one in your family; they become the "handyman", always answering the call when someone needs this or that legal documents or advice or a letter—I haven't gone back to work at a law firm, nor would I like to. No, parenting is my new career for now. Setting up a cozy home for my little Paws, trying to be the best I can as their pillar of love, strength, and courage, and the chaperone of their young aspirations. Teaching, guiding, telling stories, giving small philosophical speeches just to make a point (even if the recipient is only 4 years old staring at me wide-eyed, a bit lost, not sure whether his mamma has lost it too) dancing and singing whatever it takes. Sometimes they'll get carried away and join me, screaming at the tops of their voices, limbs and tails all over the place, and other times they will stare at me with a slightly bemused expression and then leave the room together in haste.

"It's only 7 am and we have to get out of bed and go to school; you can't be singing so early".

"Why not? It's a lovely day, and anyway, you know you don't have to go to school if you don't feel up to it".

Yes, I am one of those who believe that young creatures should be able to choose a "school-free day" every now and then if that is necessary for their well-being. After all, they are growing up so fast—leaving behind their younger versions at the end of every passing day. A "free school day" is in fact a holiday for me. A whole day with my precious two little Paws.

I suppose there will be those who will say it's understandable why with our situation—I am getting there soon—I behave the way I do, but I like to think

I am who I am regardless of the circumstances, that the reality of my life hasn't paved my way forward but rather the opposite. The way I see it, those particular circumstances were sent to me because of who I am. Nothing will stop me on my journey to fulfillment. I take my parcel willingly and do the best I can, but it must be done on my terms, my way.

While we all need our tribes around us and a sense of belonging, I was always a bit different, even as a child, as far as my dreams were concerned. I needed the love and protection of my family and friends, of course, but my dreams took me further away from everything I knew, and at an early age I understood that life is like an ocean of choices and that there are so many of them, as far as the horizon goes and beyond. Like in the ocean; you can't always see the surface, but you can never be mistaken as you are the maker of your journey. While most of my friends and acquaintances have stayed around or not so far off, my dreams have taken me on a faraway journey and here I am today, halfway through looking forward to our future adventures and challenges, holding my two little Paws on each of my sides.

How grateful I am to my dear parents who have allowed and encouraged me to dream and create my own unique path, and even though I am a mother myself now, they continue to do so every single day. It is my turn now to pave the way for my little Paws, laying down the milestones, whispering ideas and wishes in their tiny little ears as we make our way against the big and sometimes scary waves, soothing their minds and spirits after a big storm, singing a lullaby to fill up their hearts and minds with so much love to protect and encourage them on their individual journeys long after I am gone, so they too will make their dreams reality.

The birth of a lion and goddess Kali Kalita

Leopaw was born two years after Mr. Daddypaw and I got married, beautiful strong, and ever-curious. Kalipaw arrived five years later. A real goddess, strong-willed and very much opinionated, "must do everything I say at the exact moment I say" or else…. They came and took over our lives completely as if they had a magic stick swirling both of us in an everlasting ride on a magical "Merry go round". Now more than a decade has passed since embarking on our journey as parents it somewhat feels as if we are moving much faster.

Although I am used to doing multiple tasks no longer being shaken by "Merry's" paced, it does seem a bit unfair to me now both Paws are grown up that I am still constantly being tested for what feels like my acrobatic skills plus my physical and mental strength and stability while those two naughty Paws are staring at me with delight from the comfort of the sofa while I am executing their respective commands without falter.

"Ohrr will you please put down your "magic sticks" for a second and give me a hand! I am not Cinderella's godmother fairy ?!" Opps it went out of my mouth a little louder than I planned.

"I know it is important for you both to know your Mammapaw is perfect and the most capable, most deserved, and cleverer than the rest of the mammas in the whole universe and that I must score the highest points at any given test or mission you both are presenting me with. However, as grateful as I am to be your mother I must tell you that I am getting old as we speak and it is not as easy as it used to be. If you will not give me some help every now and then, I might simply… drop dead. Gone. No more. Puph."

Well, well Mammapaw, that was a bit too harsh don't you think? I mean you don't want to shake their little hearts and scare them, do you? You are after all their tower of strength and confidence, your motherly love is food for their hearts and souls, you are the foundation the base…

"Yes yes I know, I know I am their base their root their infrastructure their guiding light you name it. But sometimes I am just me; a tired mother, not to say exhausted. I mean look at me where has my pretty face gone to? Where is the rest of my furry hair? And what are these annoying white strips all over? seriously who is this creature? Help!".

Bless their hearts. My little dramatic speech has worked. While I was trying to justify my behavior to my higher self both Paws were on their feet like two soldiers on a mission. Coming, going, working, clearing, dusting, loading up the dishwasher, hanging up the laundry, hoovering the carpets and tidying up their rooms, making their dinner and a cofcif (coffee) for the mamma taking me by the hand to the sofa and giving me a foot massage each Paw on each of my sides.

Oh, I am a satisfied mamma. Indeed I am. I guess I have raised them well.

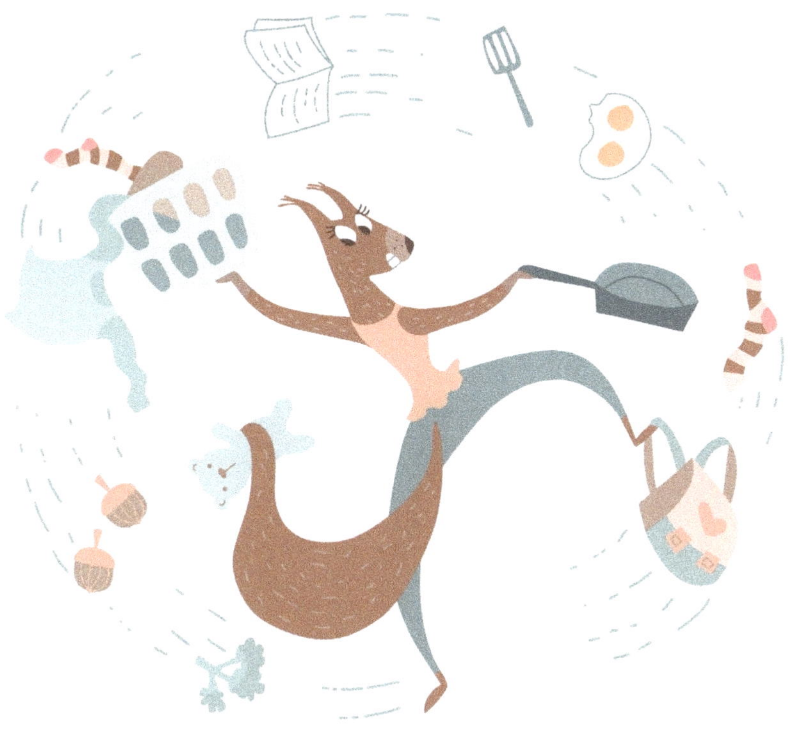

Celebrating life

"Mammapaw I have been invited to Alfred's birthday party this Friday".

"Oh my Leo that is great. When will it start do you know?"

"I shall have to find out. Oh, and there will be pizzas and cakes and all the usual birthday treats. Alfred said his parents are also taking all of us on a lantern trip in the woods. It is going to be so brilliant."

"Wow, it does sound brilliant". My head starts to pound and my mouth is getting dry. I need some coffee.

Okay, Mammapaw no need to panic it is only Wednesday today there is still time, you will think of something.

What was Alfred's mom's name?

Oh, Oh I think it's Mrs. Pixerson. Yes, Yes it is. I'll look for her on the school list... Mrs. Pittleson no... Mrs. Pudnerson no ..oh here she is Mrs. Pixerson. I shall call her straight away.

Yes, but what shall I say exactly without saying too much?... I mean I can't really ask her how many cakes there will be or what other food and treats or when they intend to serve them and can they please give me the exact time? No, I guess not. Why should anybody care about it? It might sound really awkward. Oh, God...I shall make the call now. I'll just flow with it and see what information I can get out of her.

"Hi there Mrs. Pixerson, this is Leopaw's mother speaking how are you?"

"Oh, hello good to hear from you. We are all very well thank you. How are you all?"

"Very well thanks. I am calling as Leo has told me you are celebrating Alfred's birthday with some of his friends".

"Yes it's going to be just a small group of friends oh and we are planning on taking them for a surprise treat up in the woods once the sun goes down".

"Wow, that sounds very nice indeed. Er... can I ask you a weird question ?"

"Of course. Go ahead"

"Being a birthday party and all do you plan to give special treats or food ? can you also tell me if they are going to eat before or after they go on their wood activity?"

"Oh I'm so sorry I didn't ask if you have any food allergies how silly of me, I know it is very important and can be life-threatening...".

"No, no it's okay we don't have any food allergies.. Er.. we are keeping a very strict and a healthy diet and I want Leo to be able to enjoy the birthday treats like the rest of his friends at the party, but I just need to be sure what they might be so I thought I should ask you".

That Was awkward but what can I do? Leopaw isn't ready yet to talk about it with his school friends let alone their families. Wouldn't it be so much simpler to just say "Oh, you see it is just that my Leopaw has Type 1 Diabetes no biggie"?

So many times I've thought about it. So many times I've written it. Every time my heart skips a bit. Every time it shakes me down to my core and makes me feel numb and helpless and I want to shout and scream "Why, why!" while a tornado storm gathers above my head and I can't see through it.

Breathe in, breath out, breathe in... Fresh air fills up my lungs I close my eyes and see Leo's beautiful face he is smiling at me waving his arms spreading magical oxygen into my bloodstream. I feel lightheaded and my heart expands with so much love. Love for my perfect brilliant and funny Leo the strongest of lions.

Friday has arrived and I was so nervous but pretended to be nonchalant when Leopaw arrived back from school. Lunch was waiting on the table as we had a tight schedule. It was three and a half hours before he had to leave for the party. The plan was to give the usual amount of insulin before lunch and just before Leo's departure he will get another dosage of insulin to able to eat at the party. However, Miss T1D had other plans for us. As per usual nothing is certain with her.

She likes the amusement you see she can't bear to be predictable, oh no she has a reputation to keep.

Leo's blood sugar levels were so high for no apparent reason. My heart has stopped in its place not daring to make the tiniest of noises knowing I need a few seconds to adjust and replan our next steps. Of course, my motherly instincts were telling me to keep Leo at home and forget about the party, sensing my line of thoughts Leo said he was going to the birthday party no matter what.

"Of course you are Leo, let me just fix this fiasco… what shall I give…okay I shall give you 3 units of insulin then will take another check in two hours' time, okay ?" I said as the new course of action started to take shape.

She isn't easily satisfied, Miss T1D, she needs constant action. Two hours later Leo was very low, meaning blood sugar levels were very low from Hyper to Hypo. We had 30 minutes before the party was about to begin. Now what? If I'll let Leo go there is a risk he will stay low and it is too dangerous. On the other side if he goes and eats birthday treats – which he will – without a proper cover of insulin – which I can't give when he is low – he will be high again. No matter how I looked at it the result was too risky.

For God's sake, it's only a birthday party, why does it have to be so bloody complicated!

Leo was about to cry with frustration. I knew I mustn't break his spirit whatever it takes. My mind was racing against the ticking clock, the party is about to start.

"Okay here is what we are going to do. First, take a date out of the fridge and eat it. Miss Pixerson has said you are going to eat pizzas before the trip to the woods which is planned at dusk time, not too long now, so the date will help level up your blood sugar and stop the Hypo until you eat pizza. Now listen carefully, when you finish eating the second slice of pizza text me with your phone I'll stay around Alfred's house, you will then asked to be excused for a second go outside and meet me in the car where I shall give you a dosage of insulin enough to cover two slices of pizza and a bite of the birthday cake. Sounds good?" I asked.

"Sounds great Mamma" said a very merry Leo a big smile spread on his face.

"Oh and Leo take another date and some chocolate in your bag, just in case" I said feeling restless and somewhat irresponsible.

Our plan has worked out perfectly. Leo went to the party and 20 minutes later after eating his pizza and a few other treats came out for his injection in my car. He has promised to check his blood levels two hours later and text me their results. As he has done.

Three and a half hours after he has left for the birthday party Leopaw has arrived back home happy as can be sharing his adventures with excitement. Watching him so happy and content has filled me up with so much love and joy and shook away any negative thoughts. It was the right thing to do, sending him to the birthday party. It could have been easier if we didn't have to maneuver and hide. I would certainly feel more responsible knowing there is a grownup who is watching over Leo and aware of his situation. But it was, as Leo has said, time for him to take charge and control and I agree with him. He was no longer a small child.

I shall give him the time he needs to open up and choose whoever he might want to share his medical situation with. It is his secret to tell. After all, there are still many friends and acquaintances and even family members who don't really know anything about it because I have chosen not to share it with them years ago to this very day.

Oh, and if you are curious about Leo's blood reading when he got back home it was jolly well perfect! like his mood.

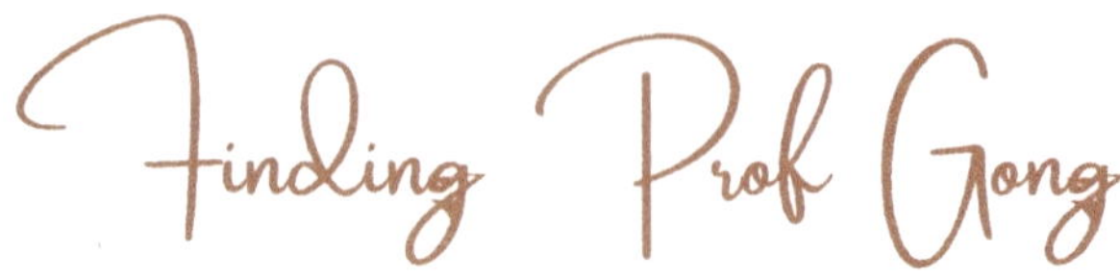

Finding Prof Gong

Two years one month and fourteen days old was our Leopaw when he was first diagnosed with T1D.

"The most straightforward diagnosis I have ever done. Don't you agree?"

"Yes… yes".

The two medical caregivers were chatting between themselves, it felt like they were given an exercise in Med school both showing off their knowledge while my head spins and the lights above have changed into a deep green and then all black.

We were taken to the ER as a matter of urgency.

"levels of blood sugar are very very high. He must be stabilized but we cannot promise anything. You have arrived a little too late".

The door was shut in my face . I could hear my Leo asking for me calling my name and my heart broke into a billion pieces. I wanted to shout and scream "give my baby back" I wanted to break that awful door get my Leo and run as fast as I can away from this nightmare. "Oh God please help my little baby please please God".

Two hours or so will go by until the door is open, this time they were asking for me.

"We are still trying to stabilize him. He isn't out of

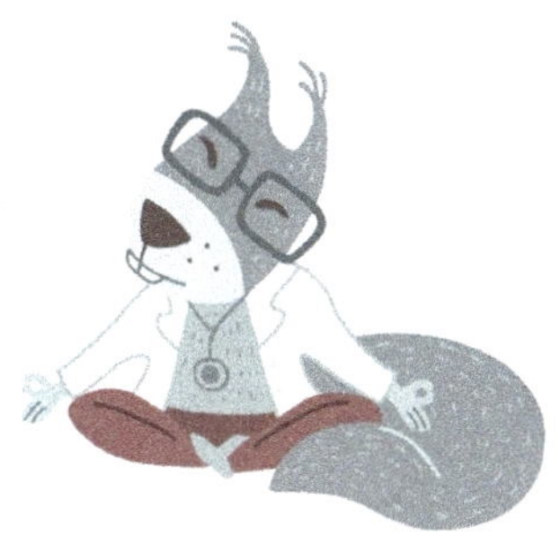

danger yet but we need you to come in and help us. Tell me immediately if you notice any difference between his pupils if they are asymmetrical this could indicate brain damage".

Another asteroid hits whatever is left of my broken body and spirit. I am surprised I am still standing. My heart pounds as I go in and I rush to see my strong brave lion. He sees me and his eyes light up he knows I am studying him carefully, he understands the seriousness on my -trying so hard - smiling face, and so he is pulling a brave face too for the sake of his Mammapaw wanting to reassure me he is fine. All will be fine. This is how very special and unique my Leopaw is. A gift from heaven kissed by the angels.

At some point they let Granny Nana in as well, by then our Leo was talking and checking out everything around him. Mr. Daddypaw was out of the country but by then was on his way back. A couple of hours later we were told we are good to leave the ER into the ward.

"Just before you leave let me tell you coming and going out of the hospital will be part of your lives from now on, be prepared".

This time it was said by an ER nurse. She knows these things or does she?

We shall see! Don't let it sink in. Don't let any of those words reach and touch you. Shut down the walls. Let these words hang up in the air until they evaporate. I refuse to let it happen. This is not going to be our way of life.

I don't wish to be ungrateful or talk badly about the way we (the adults) were treated from the moment we arrived until we left the ER, but they were not kind at all. The lot of them. Even when Leopaw was out of danger and about to leave the ER, not one kind gesture or one positive word. I know Leo was in great danger. I understand they were all under immense pressure but I think they were all very "green" and inexperienced so being sympathetic was the last thing on their list when they had to deal with complicated situations like ours. Every time the door was opened it was only to deliver "possible bad news" as if they were giving us a mental stability test and checking how deep they can push the knife in.

I don't remember if they were just training to become doctors or already doctors but I do remember the way they have treated us and it wasn't with extra kindness. Or maybe they thought we didn't deserve it, who knows.

I can't recall any of their names naturally, but as we left the ER one of them reached out to me again and said how lucky we were because if one have to have a chronic disease

T1D was it and that their hospital has one of the greatest diabetologists in the country, Prof Gong. It was a bitter-sweet thing to say to me at that point as I was still hoping our Leo will get better in a few days and it will be all gone. Those were not the words I wanted to hear but he meant well and that was the only "sympathetic" gesture we were allowed by the ER staff. We were relieved to get out of there.

Prof Gong. Prof Gong, What an unusual name. I must say I do like the sound of it, and for a split second I forget the pain and the stress and the fear as the sound of Gong rings in my head and a ray of hope sneaks in bringing a smile to my stiff pale face.

It is hard and painful to get back there even a decade after. Life and death have presented themselves as a matter of fact so intimately. When Mr. Daddypaw finally arrived, he and Granny Nana sent me home.

I still remember everything in slow motion as I was making my way back home to Woods Lane. It was hard to believe the sun was shining, birds were singing, and all living creatures were busy about their day, life goes on.

I opened the door to our quiet house with a heavy heart everything and everywhere is Leo his toys his tiny little clothes I could hear his laughter so vividly. Tears were streaming down my face as I stood in the middle of our still living room, my Leopaw is in hospital it was not just a bad dream. I must get back quickly, I said to myself making sure I'm on the move at all times knowing that if I stop just for a moment let it all sink in I will collapse. I hurried myself to the laundry room shook my tears off my face and threw my "hospital clothes" into the washing machine on the way to the shower. Suddenly I caught a glimpse of my face in the mirror in front of me. I felt ashamed and angry. A look of contempt and self-loathing for an undeserving mother was shot straight back at me like a lightning. With trembling legs, I stood there for a few seconds welcoming the pain and the guilt as the door for forgiveness was shut in front of me.

There shall be no forgiveness. Not today, not ever.

The ruling was out.

The verdict was declared.

It is your fault, Mamma. You heard the doctors, Leo was very ill when he was brought to the hospital.

How could I have let this happen?!

It is my duty to protect my baby from all harm. And I have failed.

Two doctors have seen my Leo during "that" week "*Just a virus*" or so I was told by one "*he needs some inhalation*" the other has said but I don't blame any of them. The fault is ultimately mine. I should have realized how sick he was.

I shall carry the guilt until I am no longer.

I know I am not in a position to ask for anything I accept the verdict. I have failed badly. But please God, hear me out, this I ask of you, if anything bad is going to happen to my Leo now is a good time as I go in the shower, this is your chance to strike me down. Please hear me out. I do not have the courage or the strength nor the will to stay alive should anything happen to my Leopaw.

I went in and took a long long bath.

I hope you have received my message. I mean it.

I closed my eyes and took a deep breath, unsure if my sentencing has been made yet. After a while, my eyes opened. I missed my lion terribly. Out of the shower a second later I closed the door on my way back to the hospital, leaving behind my enraged disappointed reflection.

We had eight days to let it all sink in before we were discharged. Prof Gong had to prepare the "sliding scale" – a table that indicates the right amount of insulin per different levels of sugar in the blood. We were also told we must give 30 grams of carbs in a meal but not more, Leo can only eat up to 30 grams of carbs in any given meal. A "Manuel book of operating" was also given to us, explaining when we must rush back to the hospital, and how to measure different types of food. How to treat cases of hypoglycemia and so on. That was the "easy" part though, I mean how hard can it be to calculate for example a piece of cake, a fruit salad, or a slice of pizza? Right? (wrong).

Indeed, that was definitely the easiest part because it didn't involve hurting Leo, at least not in a physical way. It got complicated when we were taught how to measure the blood with a small finger pricking which we were told we must take before every meal. It was hard enough to do at first knowing it hurts Leo pricking his tiny finger. But even that was bearable considering what must come next.

Yes, those horrible thingamies with needles. Insulin injections.

"If you want to take your baby home, you must learn how to give injections. Both of you. Maybe Granny too?" Said the diabetic nurse.

"I am not going to be able to do so. I am very sorry" said Granny.

"It's okay Granny Nana. It is understandable" I said hoping she will change her mind soon.

"I would go first. What do I need to do?" Said Mr. Daddypaw to my surprise.

Mr. Daddypaw was the first to volunteer. First, he was given an orange to practice on - An Orange! - and after he took his – literally - first shot. While the rest of us two diabetic nurses myself and Granny Nana were holding little Leopaw.

It was awful. Terrible. Leo was screaming and crying protesting the fact he was being held by four adults. Surprised to learn the pain was inflicted by his own father. I was crying too as I held his little body.

It cuts like a thousand knives let me tell you. Holding your most delicate and precious tiny 25 months old baby against his will watching him twist and turn "getting hurt" by his own parents. Every injection for every meal. I started dreading his mealtimes.

I can't do it to my little babypaw. I hate needles. I faint every time they get near me. How can I do it on my own?

"You will get the hang of it. You can stay here as long as needed until you are confident. You will be surprised, my dear. Many parents have been in your place and while it may seem impossible now I know you will be able to master it all in no time. Your baby will adapt I promise you that. You should not show weakness or sorrow. You will just treat it as a matter of fact. It is as simple as that. The more confident you get, the more confident your baby will be trusting you are doing exactly what you suppose to do".

And a master I have become. But you see I've been doing it for the last ten years as many times needed a day, I am an expert – kind of - I can give injections anytime and everywhere, whether I am fully awake or half asleep whether I am standing or sitting or lying down with a terrible flue feeling I am about to die or with an intense pounding migraine. I can give Jucsh – our own special word for "injection", somehow it sounds a bit less scary – on a Taxi ride at the exact moment the traffic light goes red, outside a school class hiding underneath my big fury coat, in a movie theatre while my two Paws are stuffing their faces with Popsiquells (squirrel popcorn). I can also give jucsh when I'm driving our car but we get stuck in a traffic jam and my Paws get hungry on the way. This is how pragmatic I have become. A new skill I have acquired and you know what I am proud of it (in a squirrely kind of way).

A message received

Seven days had gone by at the hospital and we were getting ready to go back home. Prof Gong had given us the longest list of medications and medical devices we needed to purchase before we could be discharged. I can still remember my first trip to the Pharmasquill. Tears were rolling down my face as I gave the prescriptions to the nice pharmacist. A kindhearted smiling face were staring back at me after a brief pick on the list.

"Don't worry mama everything will be okay, I promise you" said the young pharmacist.

"If only, my baby is only two years old and things are not okay…" I said.

"You see when I was two years old I have been diagnosed with Type I Diabetes too" said the pharmacist again to my great surprise.

Omg my eyes lit up as I am watching her carefully. She must be a young woman now and she looks so well and happy and everything…

"My parents have told me how hard it was when I was first diagnosed but you see I am 24 years old now and look at me, I can do whatever I want. The only thing I can recommend is for all of you to try and stay positive and happy. Ignore the "bad" readings because there might be many of them. Keeping a small child balanced at all times might be very challenging. Forget about what might be. Enjoy each moment and don't forget to smile and laugh as much as you can. This is the best advice I can give you".

An angel sent from above. I wiped away my tears and lifted my head up. I shall never forget her words. Resolved to do whatever it takes to live up to them I shook off the sadness making my way back to the hospital carrying million bags of medical supplies – just for one month.

It was time to say goodbye to Prof Gong and his staff. An eight days journey on a slippery sliding scale eyes fixed forward as we were crossing the bridge overlooking the depth underneath but very much aware of it, leaving behind on the other side the old version of our little family and as we touched the grounds again taking our first steps on an unfamiliar path a last "Thank you and goodbye wave" to the nurses and rest of the staff as they were waving back sending us away with the best wishes.

A new unknown road with many challenges ahead. We will take it step by step and hope for the best.

Going back to Woods Lane has certainly lifted our spirits.

Leopaw was thrilled and happy to be back in his own kingdom with all his toys and belongings.

Mr. Daddypaw and I gave him a big bubbly bath and afterward while both were sitting and playing it was my turn to immerse in water wash away the trauma and stress clear my head a little as I went in the bathroom avoiding meeting my face on the mirror this time, I must pull myself together think positive. A hopeful mantra in my head:

All will be well, we will be well, my baby will be well…

Talking about babies…I must say my belly does feel a bit plumped. It took a few seconds as I was starting to spin the wheels in my tired brain.

wait a minute! Now I think of it… No it can not be… can it?

Oh yes, it can. Positively clear and real.

My message Has been heard.

The judgment Has been made.

It was Life not Death.

A new life sent to me, to my lifeless numbed body, to our family.

Not only my life was sparred but an extra life was forming to make sure I would take care of myself. To keep me balanced and put a smile on my face. Sending a hopeful message while my heart cries with every prick of baby Leo's arm. To ensure I truly understand the meaning of good and bad and in between. To be thankful for what I have.

Little by little the lights were switched on inside my battered body. Thank the heavens for not being as a harsh judge as I have been. For giving me the chance to pull myself together and take matters into my own hands and charge on my new mission humbly but fiercely, grateful and forever indebted for the lives which were saved and the new ones on the way.

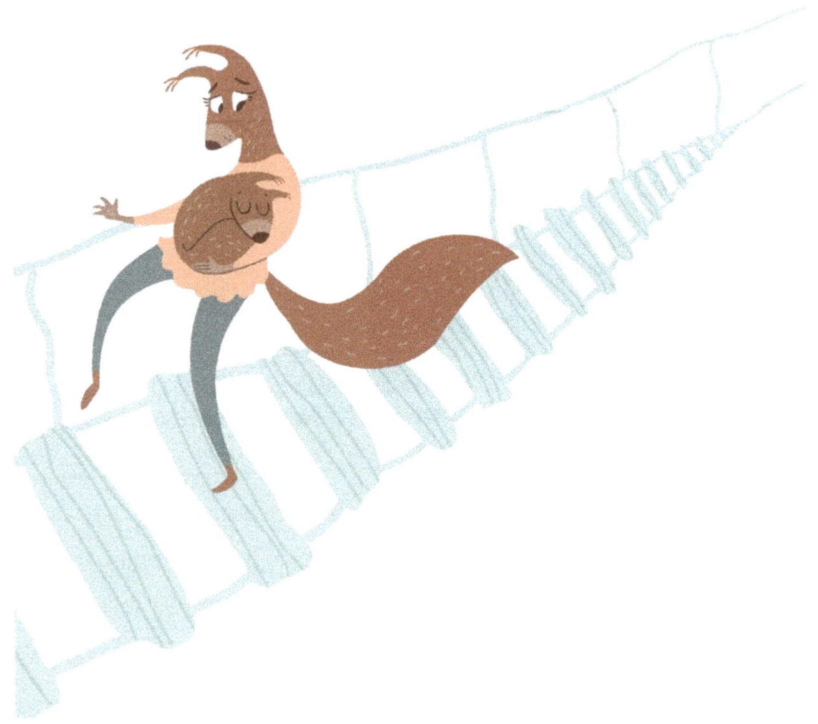

A tsunami named Kali

Like a storm, she has taken over our lives. Lovely and fluffy and definitely noisy. From the moment she has laid her eyes on Leopaw she has made sure she will never lose sight of him. Ever! She has become his twin.

Everywhere he goes she follows.

Everything he eats she eats too.

If he is sleeping she goes to sleep as well.

If he starts singing she sings louder.

If he dances she moves faster.

If he picks up a book and starts reading she wants the very same book too, ever the noble and being older Leo hands over the book to Kali and walks off to the sofa switching the TV on, and just as he sits down, as fast as lightning she is sitting right next to him singing along in her high pitched voice "Fireman Sam" while the abandoned book bangs on the floor.

Leopaw has never cried or complained about having Kali but understood she was a new member of our family. Although sometimes she can be of a nuisance to him he has learned to accept her into his life as a matter of fact and enjoy the benefits of having another mischief in the house.

You would be surprised how much noise two little squirrels could generate and when Mr. Daddypaw joins them you can actually feel the whole house trembling as the three of them scream and shout and laugh so loudly while the rest of the Wood Lane residents hurry back to their little houses puzzled covering tiny ears wishing to shield there youngest of the scarry bewildering sounds.

Oh yes, let them all know we are the Paw family we are loud and noisy and very much alive.

Having two baby squirrels in the house meant there was no time to dwell upon the past or miss it. I was busy all day long taking care of my little Paws but work would not be over for me by the end of each day. When the night comes and everyone is fast asleep my "night shift" begins and I must monitor Leopaw's glucose levels in his blood – or worse – "lack" of it. Every parent managing T1D dreads the lows – *low readings of blood sugar levels*, especially during the nights.

So many nights I have spent awake listening to the comforting peacefulness all around, watching my little Paws fast asleep wondering in their dream lands with only the moon and stars as my witnesses.

I would always put on the alarm clock just in case I fall asleep. Sometimes I could only sleep in intervals, sleep for two hours then wake up for a check, and then go back to sleep but some nights the readings will be great and I'll have the "whole" night to sleep – that is if baby Kali would permit it of course.

But there can never be a full rest for me, even when blood readings are good – on a diabetic scale of good – my mind is always busy I can never let go of the worry and just close my eyes and sleep.

I am the guardian, their keeper, I took charge of the faulty function and I must never fail again, for I have failed once and no more. There is no place for mistakes. I give all I have, and when I feel drained and exhausted I dig in deeper and deeper in search of strength.

At times it might feel like I am walking in the water against the tide or fighting a hurricane while sheltering my little Paws, but I always look for the clear blue skies I always search for the sun, and even if I stumble and falter I always find a way to stand up again for I am lucky I can give up my own strength in order to keep my little Paws safe from harm and I do it with all of my squirrelly motherly Love.

It is only when Mr. Daddypaw arrives home and takes on the night shifts when I can let go a bit and find myself again.

He is the only person I don't have to explain my feelings to, my fears and worries, my frustration and anger, and the great big love for our two little Paws as he too carries all of these feelings in his heart.

His job however takes him away from us most of the time, managing his own company SquirrSon Ltd means he must travel all over the place and so it is mostly me and the little Paws but there is one big advantage to it, it means that we are able to travel all around too for our family reunions and we do it quite frequently.

Oh dear, we just love it!

Time out of the crazy Squirrely School morning drives, no noisy Squirrdergarten -lunchtime picking ups, no rushing around the ticking clock in an effort to accomplish my daily tasks, forget about all that, and off we go to another adventure taking time off the fast daily routine in Woods Lane. Closing the door behind with gear as high as a mountain and medicinal supply enough to fill up a pharmacy we are on the way yet again to meet up Mr. Daddypaw, it is time for a break and we are all looking forward to it with much thrill and excitement.

So you see, even when it is not a holiday or a half-term break, it is our special circumstances which allow us to live especially differently. What does one thing have to do with the other you ask? Well, it does and it doesn't. I shall explain.

It is the combination of circumstances meaning; both Paws having T1D and the fact that Mr. Daddypaw is mostly away which has led me to think differently too.

We are already a family living on different terms so why not take it all the way, and make our own unique way of life. Take the hardships and challenges and combine them with a wishful thinking add to it a little bit of Paw mischief and fun and there you have it.

So far no one has objected to that, headmistresses, school counselors, and teachers, they have all expressed a favorable opinion allowing us to take some "time off" which can be up to a month every time. Their motives might be pity or compassion but I don't really mind. I hate to follow in another's footsteps and I like to pave my own way no matter how it is perceived by others. It is my way. Not only to make sure I have marked my own unique imprints but also knowing that by doing so it opens up possibilities for the unorthodox to become normal.

As I have mentioned at the beginning we are an extraordinary family. Extra crazy in the way we like to do things which are not ordinary at all.

I tell you not everyone at Woods Lane looks kindly on us but they are all a hundred percent curious!

The tree of life

As Kali approached her second year my mind started to work franticly. I dreaded her second birthday and no big plans were made for the day it was just the four of us. I have persuaded myself that if it is just going to be us giving thanks for the gift of Kali humbly and without a lavish celebration we will be spared and destiny will find someone else.

For years and years, I couldn't look at Leopaw's party pictures taken on his second birthday. Everything was normal back then, Leo was free of T1D, so tables were covered with all kinds of party treats chocolates, and cakes and all the little squirrels were happily stuffing their faces. But not this time, no we kept it simple with just a cake so Leo will not be forced to choose between the cake or the other treats. Kali was so pretty in her white tiny dress. Gorgeous, but I didn't want to think of it too much I just want her to be healthy and happy that is all I ask for my two little Paws.

The day was over without much fuss and as I was laying down to sleep I could still feel destiny hovering above.

The signs were there. Not losing weight as such but not really gaining, a little bit palish but then she was always kind of pale, she was drinking quite a lot but not overdoing it.

Do I smell Acetone? Oh, I don't know. You are starting to lose your mind, Mamma you just need to stop overthinking, Prof Gong has made it clear the chances are so very slim. I shall take little Paws to visit Granny Nana.

The little mischiefs were running and jumping in Granny's beautiful garden for hours and it was time for dinner. Leo came for his BT (blood test) and Jucsh (injection) and Kali was queuing behind him.

"Kali's turn now, me now, Kali Kalita.." pushing her tiny little finger in front of my face in determination.

"Oh Kali just move away or you might get hurt, it is not a game," I said, taken aback looking at Granny's surprised face and my heart started pounding so hard I could barely speak.

"Now Now come to Granny my little Kalita" said Granny as she kissed Kali and lifted her up to the sofa.

When my voice had finally come back to my frozen body I heard my mouth saying "This is it I am taking her to our GP tomorrow".

But there was no need to wait for a medical diagnosis I have dreaded Kali's second birthday and that milestone has arrived.

I have waited until the next morning giving us all one last night before it is official and when the morning has arrived I took Leo's extra glucometer and with a racing heart I've approached Kali who was grinning with delight, at last, she has been taken seriously.

"It might hurt a bit" I said as I pricked her tiny finger. Miss Destiny has made her choice known to the world.

With a trembling voice, I picked up my phone and called Prof Gong. At the end of our conversation, I went over to pick up Granny Nana both kids in the car on our way to the hospital and just like that we have found ourselves in the same spot yet again. Waiting for the signal not sure if or when the racing starts for the second time.

The next afternoon we were back at home. I mean I knew everything I needed to know and because it was diagnosed quite early there were no complications, no DKA (diabetic ketoacidosis) and we were allowed to go back home.

When Kali was born I also named her "my gift". Mr. Daddypaw is a proper English and insisted upon giving our Paws a few names each.

My gift she has been in many different ways.

Because Kali was used to watching Leo getting his injections without a fuss when it was her turn for injections she made sure there was no fuss too just like her older brother. This is how brave she is. Both Paws were very satisfied with the new routine. Kali because she too gets to have BT's and Jucsh like her brother and Leo because he was no longer the only one in the family who has to take on the burden of having T1D. It was only later on as Kalita was getting a bit older when she started to question why on earth must she have "*this annoying T1D?*"

I have shed quite a few tears for my second beautiful perfect baby Paw I will not lie but there was not much of a drama. In the most peculiar way, it is Kali who has helped heal my past wounds or at least helped me realize Leo's T1D was not my fault. This time there were no guilty feelings no self-inflicting pain. I was able to detect the signals I knew what I was looking for and the equation was easily solved.

This time I wasn't walking with my head on the floor feeling ashamed and unworthy while waiting for the verdict and execution. No, this time I was the mother *who has detected an early onset of T1D...* good for me. Or is it?

You see for years I have made myself believe that Leo's T1D has happened because of this or because of that and basically, it was my fault for not preventing it altogether and for not detecting it earlier as I should have. I had all the reasoning and explanations for why it has happened but then Kali's T1D arrived and in an instant they were all gone.

It was not me. It isn't something I have done or haven't done. It was due to happen anyway regardless of my actions. Or is it? I shall never know. But I do know

now that blaming myself will not help at all. At least I understand it in my head but my heart refuses to forget to forgive the young mother who has arrived at the hospital "*a bit too late*".

At the entrance to Woods Lane No.6 two trees are standing tall. Two pillars of light connecting heaves to earth. A sacred monument created with syringes and tears. Tears of pain frustration and loss, but also tears of hope and belief that the day will come and our two Paws will be free again of their respective T1D. These unique trees grow fast with every used syringe. Let us pray they will not reach the skies until that day arrives.

* Over 14,000 syringes have been used until today for insulin delivery and that is only for Leopaw. Each syringe measures 10 cm in length, if placed one on top of another their height would be the equivalent to The Burj Khalifa, The Shard and The Eiffel Tower placed on top of each other.

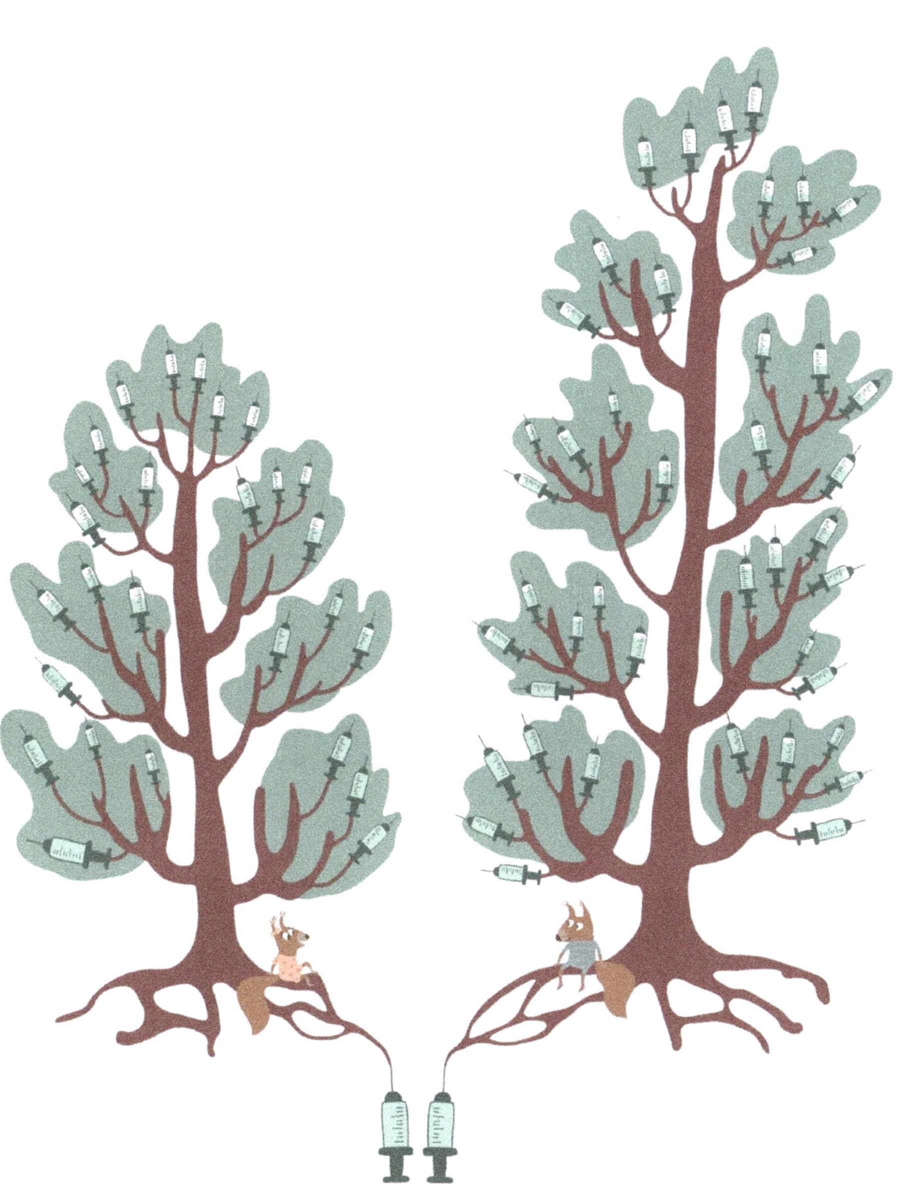

1/3 of a plate

A family member has once told me "you have a lot on your plate Mammpaw". She was referring to the fact that I have two diabetic Paws. It is true I suppose but I don't think I am different from any devoted parent taking care of her children. T1D makes it a bit more challenging, yes, but so many parents around the globe are dealing with difficult situations and terrible diseases that I am grateful for what I have, as far as one can be grateful for such things. I guess I have learned to value the words said to me when Leo was first diagnosed "If you have to have a chronic disease T1D is the one. At least you can live a normal life".

Managing T1D might be tedious at times and it has definitely taken over my personal life. Leaving me with very little time for myself, but it is a price I am willing to pay as long as my two Paws are well and happy.

Most of the time they are happy and content, I mean it is the only life they know. I suppose there is an "advantage" to being diagnosed at 25 months old. But it is not to say they are not frustrated and angry at times and just want to be "normal" like all the other kids.

It is more than understandable. I have been there myself

– but only for a short while - and I know I must let them express their feelings aloud and encourage them to do so every time they feel the need to and there have been many times Leo and Kali have felt angry and frustrated. I would be standing next to them sensing the emotions building up in the pit of their stomach, emotions they must clear out of their system and when it happens I will let it linger up in the air like a big bubble for just a couple of minutes long enough to acknowledge and respect them but when it feels right after a short while I will take out my weapon and make sure this bubble of negative emotions is destroyed.

During the first few months after Leo's T1D diagnosis, I felt I was walking on an unfamiliar ground, I took each step at a time like a blind soul unsure where will I end up next. It was impossible for me to continue like that being maneuvered, out of control. Coming up with a plan was the only way for me to get back in control, a strategic plan to win this conflict.

You can't be victorious if you declare a direct war against T1D, it is your end goal sure but you must first succumb to her endless demands, get used to being her prisoner, her toy. Let her think she has you under complete control while you study her closely and carefully until you come up with a plan. Next, you will have to gather tools and ammunition and slowly start making up your way out of her chains. The first weapon of resistance will be building up strength, mental strength.

I had the agenda all written in my head, it was my campaign against T1D. Insulin injections and blood monitoring, they are just technicalities you don't need to have special attributes in order to follow them; everyone can do that. The real challenge is completely different and I understood it straight away. In order to gain back control over his body, my first duty is to make sure Leo is mentally strong, defiant, and bold. The fact that he was only a baby when he was first diagnosed has allowed me to play a role in the shaping of his mental and physical strength.

When he was too young I knew it was up to me to become his model. I have a strong personality as it is and Leo has witnessed our family dynamics anyway. But it was not enough I had to make sure that everything around him was positive and reassuring. I had to show confidence in everything I do, the way I speak, the way I walk, and the way I interact with others. I have never let myself cry in front of him no matter how hard it was seeing his pain with every injection or with every blood drawing (which is part of his checkups), no matter how devasted I might feel about everything he must endure and fight against. My facade must be one clear of doubts or sorrow or disbelief, there is only one way for us and we shall be victorious.

In many ways, it has helped me too not to be consumed

by my sadness and fears. There was no place for them and whenever a negative thought had slipped into my head I had to crush it right there and then. If someone around me was talking about the many complications of T1D I would fire back those words into thin air. If I was to be Leo's model I had to make sure nothing could shake me, not even my biggest worries.

As Leo started to grow up it was time for teaching. Many times I have seen him watching his "strong father" with admiration and it was the perfect timing for me to make my first move. I used to sit next to him and both of us will talk about how strong Daddaypaw is and then I would introduce the idea of strength by telling him that strength comes from the mind. That if he wants to be strong he must first learn to be strong in his mind, in his heart. As the mind controls our bodies he must feel the strength running through his veins.

I had to make sure that Leo believes in himself, and that he feels content and whole with his body. I fed him the best nourishing diet body and soul. I've taught him that everything about him is special and needs special care and consideration and I have said again and again that there is nothing he can't do there is nothing he can't achieve. That for us he is the most perfect creation on earth. That he is magic, my stars, and my sun.

I have been truly blessed not only because Leo is all

of these things and more, but because I was able to achieve my goal at least the notion of it. I was able to make him realize how unique he is. It was not all easy, there were times it would be too much for him and he would sit and cry out and say that he is not as special as I think he is, but there was no place for doubts, there was no reason to doubt. Leopaw is the strongest most clever, talented funny lion but not only that — he is also very humble and kind.

Building up their mental strength was and still is goal number one for me. I know I have been talking about weapons and ammunition but my first and strongest weapon is my unconditional and total love for my children. They both know that no matter what, they are loved. They know that we believe in them, they know that anything is possible if you have the will you will find the way.

While both Leo and Kali are still young and adolescence with its many challenges is right around the corner, I think it is safe to say that both of them fully understand by now the importance of self-belief, mental strength, and resilience. They understand it is the most powerful weapon in their quest. They understand that it is okay to feel sad and frustrated and sometimes scared but also that it is up to them to make sure they don't sink into negative thoughts and move forward.

Having said that it doesn't mean that they are

completely immune to their own desires.

It was a normal afternoon and the three of us were making our way to our local "Squirrelish- Market", Kali was not more than three years old still a baby and Leo was about six years old. On our way, we were passing by a young plumped squirrel.

"Wow look how fat this kid is. He is sooo lucky" says Leo both of his eyes wide open.

"What makes you think he is lucky Leo?" I asked with surprise.

"Look at him Mammapaw he is fat! He is probably eating all day long whenever he feels like it, whatever he wants. Imagine, a chocolate cake with Pizza, a burger and chips with a bottle of Coca-Cola, a huge fruit salad as a dessert after a big meal. I mean you name it…" said an overly excited Leo.

We were all following the short round figure with our eyes until we could no longer see him. I felt instant pity for that young squirrel, it must be so uncomfortable for him. The look on Leo's face though, has made me laugh out loud. It was a look of complete admiration and awe.

So far, I think one of the most challenging aspects of having T1D for Leo and Kali is the limited portion of Carbs they are allowed to eat per every meal. At first, when they were just babies it was hard to make them eat enough carbs for their injections but as they grew older things have changed their appetite has grown with them, limiting their carbs intake has been so difficult. After all, it is in our natural instincts, feeding our children, making sure they are content. Having to be the supervisor the one who makes sure they are not eating more than they are allowed to is going against these very instincts.

It is even harder when there are family gatherings and dinner parties when they are the only ones who are restricted to a fixed amount of carbs while watching everybody else eating as much as they want, whatever they want. It was difficult for both Mr. Daddypaw and myself so initially, we have agreed not to take part in these gatherings or to arrive later on after our Paws have been fed. But as they grew older and understood more it was an essential part of their learning process, as painful as it might be, hiding from situations will not make them strong and they must face reality as it is, not by suppressing their feelings but by understanding. They have to learn to accept that it is for their own good, for their own health, and that they must take care of their bodies.

When they were small I use to say that in order to build a strong tall building you must first lay a strong infrastructure and by having a strict healthy diet they are doing exactly that. Yes, it might seem to them that the rest of us are lucky as there are no limits and we can indulge and feed our empty desires but it is only momentarily while in the long term keeping a strict healthy diet is way better and when they are old enough they will appreciate it more. The older Leo gets the stronger the sparkle in his eyes shines when I talk about having a strong infrastructure.

It may not be that easy though, there is still a long way to go, and nowadays every social gathering is all about food. It is no longer about music and dancing or similar activities, food is always the main part of the gathering. But thankfully Leo and Kali are old enough and now very much aware of their bodies. Both of them love doing sports. Kali has dance classes twice a week and she loves "*singing and dancing and K-pop. Thank you and bye*". Yes, K-pop has reached our realm too. And Leo is into martial arts, oh he loves hardcore exercises.

I must say it has been extremely helpful that Leo is a huge fan of the human footballer "legend" (as Leo would say) Christiano Ronaldo or shall I say CR7. Naturally, Leo has seen every available video and read every possible article but most importantly he has learned that his "legendary man" has a very strict diet of his own choice in order to make himself better, stronger, and healthier. So, all of the sudden it is not only the words of his sometimes over-the-top Mamma about a *strong infrastructure*, Oh no, one look at his idol and he can see the results for himself. But they don't just come for free, it takes hard work, resilience, and determination on the road to success. Why thank you Mr. CR7, for that reason alone you are and shall always be a superhero for the Paw family.

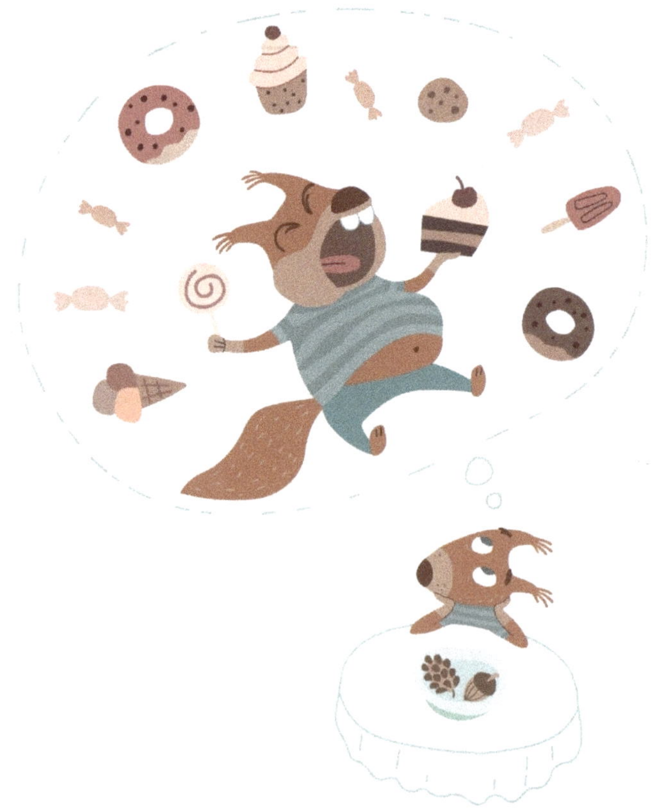

"So, the good Betta soldiers give it another try hiding away from the Killer cells moving forward determined to succeed maybe just maybe there is a chance they will make it this time…Peuchuchuchu… a violent shooting has started and they are all gone. Again" I say with an exasperated voice as I jump from side to side pretending to be the deceased soldiers.

"But why do they kill their own? I mean they are all on the same side, aren't they?" Asks a much confused Leopaw furrowing his eyebrows in an effort to find an answer.

"Yes, you are quite right my darling when we find the answer to your question we will know how to stop this silly and unnecessary conflict inside your beautiful bodies" I said.

"Puchuchu let's see you try to fight Kali Kalita," says Kalipaw as she storms in with her Nerf gun dropping on the floor pretending to finish off a Killer cell. "You're a goner". She says triumphally.

"That's right you bastard" I hear myself say without thinking, both pairs of eyes on me.

"What if there'll be a special vehicle or something like it, the Betta soldiers can be protected inside and will be able to survive the attacks," says Leo. I can feel his mind moving fast.

"It must be an armored vehicle or better yet an undetectable one," I say in frustration and suddenly I too like the poor Betta soldiers feel so helpless. I mean human beings have reached space 61 years ago. They have managed to clone animals, to build autonomous vehicles, they have developed artificial intelligence and robots, and probably all kinds of technologies we still haven't heard of. I am sure I have read somewhere that these strange humans can even book a holiday and fly themselves out to space now. With all the advances they have made why is it still so difficult to find a way around the self-immunity attack and lack of insulin? All we need is to find the restart button. To reprogram the system. To reeducate the faulty crazy killer cells and send them off to a faraway ashram so they can find their nirvana and let us all live in peace. Literally.

Obviously, I was sailing too far away with my own thoughts and for too long – as it often happens – only to find out that both Paws have left me alone and are now in their playroom completely engaged in a loud Nerf - fight both fully dressed to impress. It is a big fight indeed as the rest of the household has now become a war zone, bullets whizzing past my head both Paws are yelling with excitement as the drama continues all around.

"Be careful please, try not to break the vase... No

no, don't jump off the chandelier Leo… Kali do you know that limbs can actually break if you throw yourself so hard on the floor?!…please can you two just calm down?" I say but there is no point, they can't hear me. I better clear myself out of their way. I am too old for this. How nice it could be if someone could ship Me to a nice ashram somewhere….

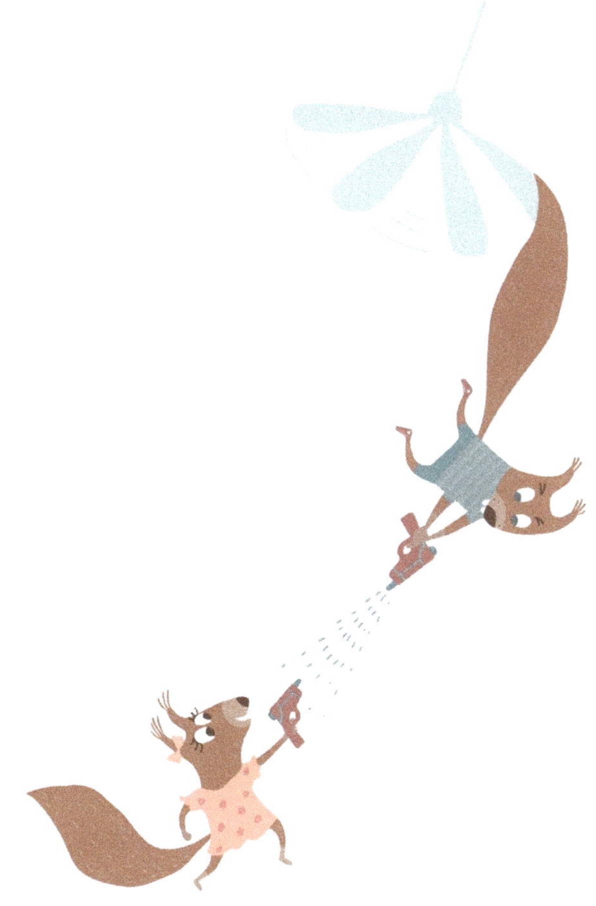

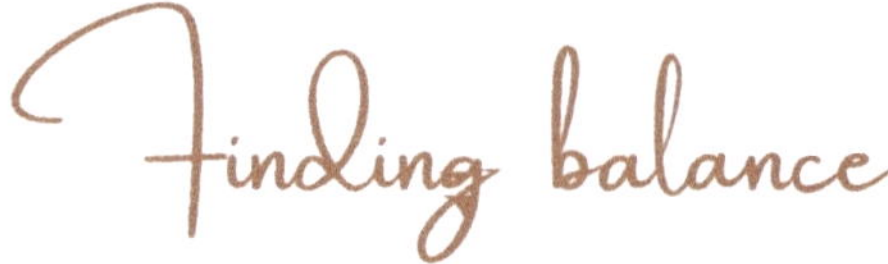

Finding balance

"What is balance?" I ask both Leo and Kali.

"Balance is having stability," says Leopaw.

"Balance is having control over your own body," says Kalipaw.

Balance is a perfect picture. Everything and everyone situated in their most outstanding way. For me, the greatest lesson in life is finding balance. If only we all had a magical stick to help us find and regain balance. Like a campus to direct us when we are lost at sea or on land.

Many times I've been asked what is the true meaning of diabetes to me. My answer is quite simple. Finding balance.

Everything needs to be balanced every aspect of our lives, every aspect of our personalities, our desires. Our bodies must work in a perfect balance every organ must give its share, there must be a perfect harmony at all times and we must adapt to every change and embrace it swiftly. Our mindsets must be fine-tuned and adjusted accordingly.

Now how do you achieve it is a different question and most of us will agree it is nearly an impossible mission.

It is even more so when T1D is part of your life. Most

will say T1D is about keeping blood sugar balanced. But that is only partially correct. Leveling blood is the end result of the equation. It is the road to get there which will try you again and again. It is Miss T1D with her infamous reputation. You will be in her hands like a marionette and she will play and manipulate you until she takes complete control over your own existence and you will find yourself thinking about her all day all night. She will be your beginning and your end like a poisonous lover.

It has taken me quite a while to understand it. At first, I was hit badly and refused to shake it off me. I've been deeply immersed within the loss. Loss of my baby's perfect health. It was so hard that even breathing was an unbearable task for me, not medically but I was in so much pain coming into terms with the new reality that I refused to accept it. I refused to surrender to the new forced circumstances. I thought if I kept breathing freely it means I have accepted the new conditions and I couldn't contemplate it at the time. It was like there were walls around my mind and they were blocked and heavily secured by my own mini guards. The only thing I would allow in was the wishful thinking that Leo will be cured in a matter of days or weeks at the most, anything else was utterly unacceptable. I was terrified and felt so helpless and scared I had to believe things were going back to the way they used to be very soon.

But like Miss T1D's own set of rules, life has her own way of fashion, and little by little you start getting used to it taking every day as it goes and learn to breathe in between, and soon days turn into months turn into years and there you are a decade later. A bit wiser, a bit calmer, and extremely good with needles!

When realization strikes you understand that you too have chosen Life. Living is your first priority. Yes, Miss T1D is part of it but you will not give her all of you. Yes, she will continue to play the unpredictable and you will continue to fail miserably again and again and even if you believe you have finally found the correct algorithm it will soon explode right in your face leaving you shocked and confused and completely deflated. But you will find your strength and rise again and one day you will understand that it doesn't have to be a "perfect" balance it is enough if there is Some kind of a balance and you will find yourself smiling, so busy you will be so immersed in life, you will forget she is there at times.

It is where I stand today, at this moment in time. A decade of experience raising two magnificent creatures. My two sweet brave funny and magical Paws and in our shadows walks Miss T1D, behind. There might be times she will try to lift up her head again, oh but we know how to handle her. She will not break us, she will not take the smile off our faces. Never.

Ever since they were very young I have taught Leo and Kali that life is a journey of self - discovery a journey we must walk with our best equipment and knowledge, it is a journey that can never be rushed until it takes its course. It is up to us to make it adventurous and exciting and we must learn to overcome obstacles and achieve our goals, reach our destinations and fulfill all of our dreams. With hope that someday along the way they will lose Miss T1D forever.

I pray that day will come during my lifetime and I shall witness both my Paws free of her chains. But even if it won't arrive during my time I know it is because of T1D both of them are mentally strong, mature, and more than capable to endure her challenging management. At times they might feel angry and frustrated but at others, she will go unnoticed.

Whatever happens, there is still a way to go, there are lives to live and we must make the best of it. Waking up every morning to a new day, watching my two Paws growing up, enjoying their wisdom their wit and humor, their talents and unique personalities just being part of their lives fill me with renewed energy and excitement, and most of all lots of love and appreciation for these two extraordinary souls, two powerful sources of life who have both chosen me above all others to be their mother. I shall do whatever it takes to be worthy of them.

We have come so far. We have been through a lot.

My eternal love will always light up their ways as they figure out their special unique lives.

"Good night Mammapaw" Mr. Daddaypaw has just sent me a message.

I must have been mesmerized by the fire as I find myself snuggled up in my rocking chair with my yellow pom poms throw. It is quite late and I must make my way to bed. Both Leo and Kali are sleeping and it is time for last BT and afterwards hopefully a full night's rest for me.

I go first to Leo's room and find him fast asleep. On a shelf next to his bed lay both of his tiny boxing gloves. He is so enthusiastic about Thai Boxing that he can't leave his gear out of his bedroom. When he was first registered his coach called me and introduced himself. The first thing he had said to me before I could even mention T1D was that all of his students must keep a very healthy diet. I was speechless and my head went like *are you kidding me...would you like me to tell you about having a strict diet...!*

You see, for the first time in his life having a strict diet is a must not because of his T1D but because of the hobby he likes so much. Leo can now start to enjoy the fruits of his efforts.

It seems like the pieces are falling into the right places.

Bless my boy. Sleep safe and sound. A goodnight kiss.

Next, I go to Kali's room. It seems she has worked a bit and put some order in her messy room. All piles of clothes are now gone. I have a pressing feeling that they were merely moved from her room into the laundry room. I shall deal with it in the morning.

On her table is a picture of her current K-drama star. She keeps changing them on a weekly basis. It makes me smile and more so when I think of Mr. Daddypaw's reaction when Kali has informed him that she has a "boyfriend… Oh don't worry father I know all about romance because I am a romantic girl".

Poor Mr. Daddypaw his eyes nearly popped with horror. "You are not even 10 years old Kali and since when do you call me Father ?.."

Needless to say that the boyfriend is an imaginary one, well not completely imaginary as we all see his face hanging all over her bedroom walls. Not to worry though, within a week or so a new image will be decorating her walls. After all, she is goddess Kalita and nothing in the world can stop her from doing exactly what she wants!

Bless my girl. Sleep tight. A goodnight kiss and off I go to my own bed. BT's were good so I can sleep all through the night.

I can hear the wind banging on the windchimes outside like an orchestra conductor. I look at two tree branches dancing outside my window.

Isn't it great being part of this glorious creation?! Soon birds will be singing as the sun climbs above the clouds. With her long loving arms, she will embrace and bless us all with a new beautiful day.

Tears of joy and hope are streaming down my face as I think with excitement and gratitude of the journeys ahead.

xxx

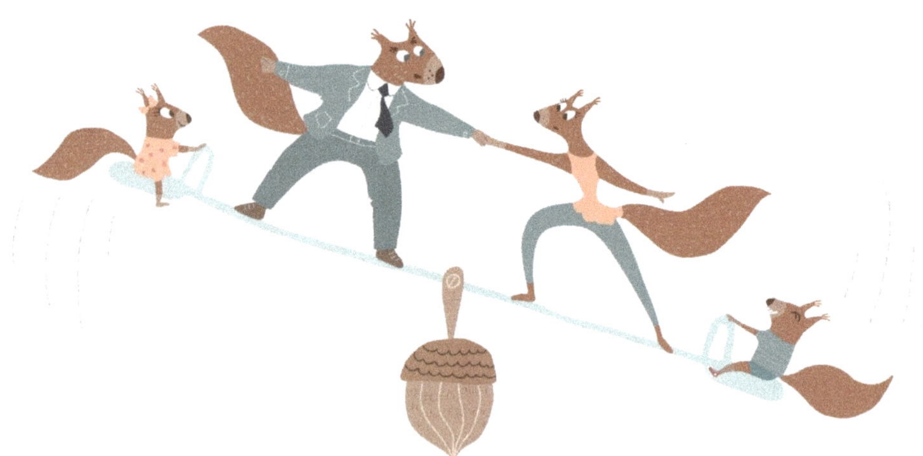

Epilouge

It has been a hectic couple of months. We have spent the summer holiday in Spain and Portugal then back home on September for school. Since Leo's birthday is also on September we took a short trip to London in order to celebrate it properly. St. James park was so gorgeous with it's autum leaves.

Now November is just around the corner but I still haven't recovered from all the travelling. I'm constantly tired and haven't been able to sleep very well for quite a while now. If I'm ready to admit it I have lost some weight too but what worries me most is the fact that lately I have started drinking too much water, like a lot of it. In fact in one day I drink more than I would drink in a month !!!

It's all too overwhelming. I have been here before.

I feel shiverish.

Shall I call Prof Gong?

I am going to call Prof Gong…

Acknowledgments

My most talented and extremely busy dear friend/sister Mrs D. Robinson for bringing this book into life. Thank you for taking this project to your heart. Ms. Anna Solemani for editing and proofreading. Ms. Maria Dronfort for wonderful illustrations, working with you has been a sheer joy. The real Mr. Daddypaw for dreaming the dream of our two extraordinary littlepaws; even though we were oceans apart. My own Mama for your unconditional love and support. You are our cure God bless you! The real Prof. Gong you are one of a kind. Sorry for making you feel restless at times. My two sisters, SK and IB your love and support means the world to me. Every minute spent with you fills my heart with joy and magic. Thank you for being the best unties in the world! My Dad and my Granny I miss you both every second of every day. My two older brothers growing up with you has made me who I am in spirit and heart. You are the best! Lastly, my precious littlepaws my heroes; AR and AS you are my shining stars. Thank you for letting me share your story. There is no end to my love and gratitude when it comes to you. God bless you!

9 781803 698793